Praise for *Yoga for Healthy Knees*

Yoga for Healthy Knees is a highly readable and practical guide for those seeking information about safe yoga practice for their knees. A must-read for anyone interested in knee rehabilitation and for yoga teachers, too.

—Cybèle Tomlinson, codirector of the
Berkeley Yoga Center; author of *Simple Yoga*

Sandy Blaine's *Yoga for Healthy Knees* is doubly interesting. It describes how she overcame her own knee pain using yoga poses. It also teaches the reader about safe movements and specific poses that can protect and improve their own knees as well. I recommend this book for its clarity, organization, and positive attitude of healing.

—Judith Hanson Lasater, Ph.D, P.T., yoga teacher; author of
30 Essential Yoga Poses: For Beginning Students and Their Teachers

Yoga for Healthy Knees

Rodmell Press Yoga Shorts Series

Yoga for Pregnancy by Judith Hanson Lasater, Ph. D., P.T.

Yoga for Healthy Knees by Sandy Blaine

Yoga Abs by Judith Hanson Lasater, Ph. D., P.T.

with more to come . . .

rodmell press

YOGA SHORTS

YOGA

FOR HEALTHY KNEES

WHAT YOU NEED TO KNOW FOR
PAIN PREVENTION AND REHABILITATION

▼　▼　▼　▼　▼　▼　▼　▼

Sandy Blaine

RODMELL PRESS　　BERKELEY, CALIFORNIA, 2005

To those who have passed on the gifts of yoga throughout millennia: my yoga teachers—past, present, and to come—and to their teachers.

▼　▼　▼　▼　▼　▼　▼　▼

Yoga for Healthy Knees: What You Need to Know for Pain Prevention and Rehabilitation, copyright © 2005 by Sandy Blaine. Photographs by David Martinez. All rights reserved.

No part of this book may be reproduced or transmitted in any form or by any means, electronic or mechanical, including photocopying, recording, or by an information storage or retrieval system, without written permission from Rodmell Press, 2147 Blake St., Berkeley, CA 94704-2715; (510) 841-3123, (510) 841-3191 (fax), www.rodmellpress.com.

Library of Congress Cataloging-in-Publication Data is available.

Printed in China
First Edition
ISBN 1-930485-08-5
10 09 08 07 06 05　2 3 4 5 6 7 8 9 10

Editor: Linda Cogozzo
Copy Editor: Katherine L. Kaiser
Indexer: Ty Koontz
Lithographer: Rockaway / Phoenix Asia

Cover and Text Designer: Gopa & Ted2, Inc.
Cover, Interior, and Author Photographer: David Martinez

Distributed by Publishers Group West
Text set in Dante

Contents

▼ ▼ ▼ ▼ ▼ ▼ ▼

Acknowledgments

▼ ▼ ▼ ▼ ▼ ▼ ▼ ▼ ▼ ▼ ▼

I am so excited and grateful to have had the opportunity to write my first book. I have many people to thank for helping me bring this work to life.

First and foremost, I thank publishers Donald Moyer and Linda Cogozzo at Rodmell Press for their support and guidance along the way. In addition, Donald has been one of the primary teachers in my life. I thank him for teaching me that yoga in the style of B. K. S. Iyengar is a mindfulness practice, and for mentoring me throughout the years with a generosity of spirit that I will always be grateful for.

Many other wonderful yoga teachers have guided me along the way. What I have learned from each has contributed to shaping my own evolving practice and this book. In particular, I appreciate Amy Cooper, John Friend, Judith Hanson Lasater, Tim Miller, Jill Edwards Minye, Leigha Nicole, Sarah Powers, Erich Schiffman, and Mary Lou Weprin.

I gratefully acknowledge Wendy Lichtman, my wonderful writing teacher. In addition, I appreciate all the women and fellow writers who have been in her writing groups with me. I have participated in Wendy's classes on and off for several years, and the list of writers in these groups is too long to name here. Know that I carry your stories and lessons with me. I especially thank Joan Steinau Lester for sharing her time and editing skills as I worked on various writing projects throughout the past few years.

Thank you to my dear friend and wordsmith extraordinaire, Clive Chafer, for his support, contributions, and last-minute brain-storming.

Thank you also to Judith Hanson Lasater and Cybèle Tomlinson, who were the book's first readers outside of the publishers, for their support, insight, and contributions.

I express my gratitude to those whose work you see in these pages: photographer David Martinez, for his beautiful work; model and yogini Deborah Ramelli, who is also both my friend and my teacher; editor and producer Linda Cogozzo; makeup artist France Dushane; caterer Jeff Mason; photographer's assistant (and wall supporter) Charlie Nucci; production assistant Star Griffin; studio manager Aneata Hagy; and last but not least, Dice, the Wonder Dog, for his uplifting presence. All of you made it such a supportive and successful day.

I appreciate Hugger-Mugger Yoga Products and Marie Wright Yoga Wear, who generously donated their props and their clothing, respectively, to the photo shoot.

My heartfelt thanks go to my business partner, Betsy Weiss, the codirector of the Alameda Yoga Station. From Betsy, I have learned so many invaluable lessons about teamwork and the meaning of partnership. Without her, there would be no Alameda Yoga Station, the place in our little corner of the world where I have been most able to explore the path of teaching and to make a living in a way that (I hope) gives back more than it takes from the world.

And most important, I acknowledge the many students who have come to my classes throughout the years. Thank you for allowing me to share my practice with you and for being my most inspiring teachers.

Introduction

▼ ▼ ▼ ▼ ▼ ▼ ▼ ▼ ▼ ▼ ▼

I never expected to be a yogi, to have a serious yoga practice, or to write this book. I originally showed up at yoga class on a whim, simply searching for some kind of exercise I could enjoy without doing further damage to my injured knees. I was prone to knee problems due to fairly common congenital musculo-skeletal patterns; these problems had been exacerbated by the dance and tumbling classes that I loved as a child. The result of this combination was that, by my early twenties, I suffered from multiple traumatic injuries that had left me in chronic pain.

Protecting my knees and being physically limited for a lifetime was a daunting prospect. I had gone through extensive physical therapy, such as it was in the early 1980s, with limited results. So I never dreamed that profound healing was available through yoga. I was amazed to discover that within six months of regular practice, my knee pain had disappeared.

Although glimpses of my old knees resurface from time to time (if I'm very tired or miss too many days of practice), the stability and relief that therapeutic yoga, as developed by B. K. S. Iyengar, author of *Light on Yoga,* brought to my traumatized knee joints was nothing short of miraculous. Out of a mixture of curiosity about how this came to be, and deep gratitude that it did, I began a study of yoga that has become a serious journey.

Yoga works. When practiced therapeutically, yoga brings the individual joints and the overall body into balance in two primary ways. First, moving through a variety of asana (yoga poses) stretches and lengthens tight muscles, and strengthens lax ones. As a result, the joints have an increased range of motion and greater structural support.

Next, and equally important, skeletal alignment is important in Iyengar-style yoga, which teaches the body to bypass its habitual patterns and learn new ones, rather than moving along the path of least resistance. How does this work? Consider how grooves are worn into a rock by a continuous stream of water flowing along the same path, and how that pattern would change if the flow were routed along a different path or several paths. With the joints, the bones are pulled toward the tight muscles. If some muscles are very tight, the bones can be subtly, but continually, pulled out of alignment. Over time, this causes joint wear and tear that results in chronic aches and pains or more serious conditions.

Many people believe they have flat feet, which is a congenital anatomical condition, when, in fact, they have weak or collapsed arches, which is muscular and can be corrected through exercise. In my case, I had naturally weak arches and inner ankles, which led to underdeveloped inner quadriceps and a tendency for the strong outer quads to pull my kneecaps toward the outsides of my legs. It's a common pattern and people with both conditions often develop knee pain. Eventually, extreme stress on one of my joints (due to an unfortunate landing on a trampoline) pulled a patella (knee cap) out of alignment. This excruciatingly painful experience left me with slack, weak ligaments that no longer did their job of holding the bones in place. After a while and after multiple injuries, it didn't take much stress to dislodge the knee.

My first years of yoga practice were challenging, as I made many discoveries about my own physical patterns through practicing standing poses, which I initially found, well, torture. The underdeveloped muscles of my feet and inner legs screamed with protest, but my intuition told me that it was worth continuing. And I couldn't refute the evidence of how wonderful I felt, physically and mentally, after each class. My own yoga students often giggle when I talk about the difference between sensation and pain, but come quickly to realize that the body's natural wisdom easily makes the distinction. With just a little practice, most of us can discern pain—the body's clearest signal that something is wrong—from the healthy muscular sensations caused by strengthening and stretching underused or overworked muscles.

After some months of regular practice, it dawned on me that my experience of my knees had dramatically shifted—for the better. Without my noticing, yoga practice had stretched out my tight hips and outer quads, built up muscle around the inner knee, and brought more awareness and balance to my feet and my ankle joints. And suddenly, I wasn't waking up in the morning with painful, vulnerable knees. The standing poses became gradually easier and, even more gradually, my psychology regarding the trauma of my knee injuries also shifted, so that I wasn't walking so gingerly and approaching daily life with such caution. Yoga allows me to experience the movements of daily life with more freedom and enthusiasm, and it is this profound gift that I hope to share with you through this book.

How to use this book. As I look back on my experience, I am convinced that yoga can help each person to discover his or her body's own natural wisdom and utilize it to realize greater healing. I am not an expert on every type of knee injury, but I have a great deal to share about what worked for me. Everyone's body is different, so it may be that my program won't be exactly right for you. However, it is my hope that my ideas about yoga and knee rehabilitation will, at least, yield enough information and clues that, with experimentation, you can adapt this program in the way that best meets your own needs.

In all honesty, therapeutic yoga practice takes a fair amount of kinesthetic intelligence, or body awareness, and mindfulness. It's not possible to heal from within unless you are paying more attention to what is actually happening than to what outside sources tell you "should" be happening. And developing a regular practice of any kind requires a tremendous amount of dedication and discipline. The good news is that both can be learned. Just as any aptitude can be cultivated, physical intelligence increases with practice. And pain or restricted movement are great motivators to keep practicing.

The next part of this book talks in more detail about various knee conditions and gives some guidelines for practicing. I encourage you to pay attention to the guidelines and not simply jump ahead to the practice section. Mindfulness is a key element of yoga and is particularly important when practicing therapeutically. Practicing by rote or without proper attention can actually be harmful. Yoga students are sometimes told that their injuries are gifts or lessons, a sentiment that often evokes eye-rolling frustration. But I arrived at yoga certain that avoiding another painful knee injury was far more important to me than achieving any of the poses, and this was a great starting point. I never expected to do certain poses, such as Padmasana (Lotus Pose) or Virasana (Hero's Pose, Figure 12A), so I had no reason to push. And in retrospect, I realize that was in large part what kept me safely on the road to healing, rather than exacerbating my condition. To this day, I am careful about never doing anything in my practice that causes pain. If you incorporate only one idea from this book into your own rehabilitation, I suggest that be the one.

Following the practice guidelines are instructions for the seventeen poses that I consider to be the most essential ones for knee therapy, plus some variations to adapt them for individual bodies. These poses take the body, particularly the lower half, through the most important range of motion for strengthening and stretching the muscles around not just the knees, but also the feet, ankles, legs, and hips, each of which has its own particular relationship to how the knees function. The photographs and instructions are meant to serve as a guide. The poses themselves are best learned from a well-qualified instructor, who can see what you are doing and guide you until you can feel for yourself from the inside when your alignment is healthy and correct. The asana section of this book, which should be used as an adjunct to this personal attention, provides some general instructions for helping to learn each pose, as well as specific points to focus on in order to derive maximum therapeutic benefit from a pose.

Following the asana section are suggested asana sequences to practice. A fact of yoga is that it is not a quick fix: yoga must be practiced regularly over time in order to yield results. And in order to maintain those results, practice must be kept up rather than dropped when satisfaction is achieved. A therapeutic practice is most effective when followed daily or almost daily, but the reality of modern life is that most of us don't have a free hour every day to devote to a new activity. Although I believe that our lives would be happier if we could all slow down and take far more time out for caring for ourselves, practicality asks us to simply do what we can. So, to start with, do the full practice as many days of the week as you can manage. When it isn't possible to do the full practice— and later, once you are practicing for maintenance—use the shorter sequence in this section. It is always more effective to do a few poses with quality of attention and relaxed breathing than to rush through in an attempt to fit everything into a short time. And perhaps that's a lesson we can take with us when we leave the yoga mat, incorporating it into the other areas of our lives.

With that in mind, the next section of this book addresses knees in daily life. Although I can't speak to every single situation that your body is in throughout the day, there are a few particularly important areas, such as exercise (or lack thereof), where your knees would benefit from more attention to your choices, and I've tried to give some information to help with this process. However, you are always the best source of knowing what is good for you. If you notice one of your regular activities (such as driving a stick shift car or skiing), doesn't seem to be having a good effect on your knees, I urge you to pay attention to your own perceptions and see what changes you can make. Resistance to change often arises out of denial, that is, the wish to hang onto the way things used to be or how you wish they were. As you proceed with this book, try to keep an open mind about making changes. Change is inevitable, and my own experience is that it is often positive, especially when you choose it consciously. Miracles are available, but most often they are the ones that we create ourselves, step by conscious step.

Part One

Factors in Common Knee Problems

▼ ▼ ▼ ▼ ▼ ▼ ▼ ▼ ▼ ▼ ▼ ▼ ▼ ▼ ▼ ▼ ▼

M ANY KNEE PROBLEMS are the result of a combination of congenital patterns and external stress, meaning, how the body moves in response to those patterns. Natural laws are powerful, and the path of least resistance has a great deal of influence on how the body develops and ages. For example, chances are you always, every single time, use your looser arm to reach behind your back to scratch an itch or do up a zipper. Unless you're consciously thinking about it (and why would you be?), you'll almost certainly reach with the arm that moves more easily. So the tighter shoulder joint is not asked to stretch, and, with age and underuse, continuously loses mobility. In this way, your natural imbalances are reinforced and exacerbated over time, causing many of the aches and pains associated with middle age.

Hyperextension. Most garden-variety knee problems are due to multiple factors. Hyperextension, for example, occurs when the knee joint is overly flexible and the tibia moves past the femur in extension, instead of the two bones stacking directly one on top of the other, as with healthy extension. When in hyperextension, the leg extends too far and moves past the point of being straight. Hyperextension can also be functional, meaning, rather than being born with it, you develop it by habitually locking the knees.

Feet: supination and pronation. The foundation of any physical structure is crucial to its integrity, and with the human bodies, the foundation is the feet.

The feet function best and provide the healthiest foundation for the rest of the body when the arches are strong and the "four corners" of the feet are in balance. Much the way that the tires of your car need to be balanced and aligned in order for the car to function efficiently, balance in the feet affects the entire structure of the body, from the ground up. Few of us have perfectly balanced feet: it is far more common to tend toward either supination (usually found in those with higher arches) or pronation (associated with flat or collapsed arches), which means that one side of the ankle will also be underdeveloped and the other side will be correspondingly overdeveloped from supporting more than its share of weight. A pattern like this runs from the ground up the entire body, just as the Leaning Tower of Pisa leans off to the side (and will eventually fall over and collapse completely) as a result of just a small miscalculation in the supporting stones at the very bottom. And, just as with a building or a car, the imbalances you start with lead to developmental problems, such as instability or poor tracking of the joints caused by subtle but chronic misalignment. These may be hardly noticeable until middle age, but worsen over time and at some point begin to accelerate. A very common knee problem, for example, is the uneven wearing of the meniscus (the cartilage under the kneecap) caused by a knee joint that is out of balance in just this way; eventually, one side wears down significantly enough to create discomfort, and may even produce arthritis of the knees.

Tight muscles. Simple tight muscles can also bring about joint pain and injury. Joints cannot be healthy unless the muscles that support them are, and healthy muscles are both strong and supple. Prevention is always more effective than any cure, and this is especially true with joint problems, because ligaments, once torn or stretched out of shape, do not heal. Tight outer hips and hamstrings both put undue stress on the knee joints, and both age and athletics will inevitably cause these muscles to tighten (albeit the quality of aging muscles is somewhat different depending on whether they are tight due to neglect or overuse); the combination of the two is almost poisonous unless countermeasures are taken. Generally, we don't realize that we are losing range of motion until it is already substantially reduced; this loss is, in large part, preventable through regular stretching. Flexible muscles and free range of motion are associated with youth, and although it is true that they take more time and effort to maintain as we get older, enduring physical energy and youthfulness are the payoffs that make the expenditure worthwhile.

Part II

Practicing Yoga for Knee Care

▼ ▼ ▼ ▼ ▼ ▼ ▼ ▼ ▼ ▼ ▼ ▼ ▼

Guiding Your Practice

YOGA IS A UNIQUE DISCIPLINE that can be many different things to different people. It is neither physical therapy nor simply exercise; but it can be used in either of these ways and it does incorporate elements of both. To use asana (yoga poses) effectively as a therapeutic practice, mindfulness is essential. As you practice, you are getting to know yourself, a fundamental component of yoga practice. B. K. S. Iyengar's philosophy recognizes that you can't know yourself on a spiritual level if you aren't conscious in your body. From the point of view of healing, learning how to best nurture yourself with asana requires attentiveness and a certain amount of experimentation. In this section, I outline a few key points to pay attention to in your practice; they will facilitate healing and also develop awareness. And it is awareness that makes for a safe and intelligent yoga practice.

Do not practice yoga poses that hurt your knees. Pain is your body's signal that something is wrong. While in some poses, you may experience mild sensation in the ligaments that stretch over the kneecaps. But the operative word here is "mild." Approach each asana gently, even if you know the pose. Avoid or modify any asana that creates pain in the knees. Remember, not every body is meant to do every pose: accept yourself as you are. Your abilities will certainly expand with regular practice, especially if you work with sensitivity and care.

Learn the difference between the sensation of stretching and actual pain. Pain in the knee is joint pain, which is always to be avoided. In some poses, however, you will feel intense sensation in your leg muscles, either from the work of stretching or the demands of strengthening those muscles as they work in new ways. You can easily learn the difference between healthy sensations and harmful ones by listening to your body. Notice how you feel when you come out of an asymmetrical stretch or pose: does your body call out to do the same stretch or pose on the other side? This is your body recognizing a healthy movement and striving for balance. Your body, however, will always try to avoid pain. On the one hand, you can breathe through intensity and the body will become stronger and more open; trying to endure pain, on the other hand, is likely to cause or deepen injuries.

Use your quadriceps muscles to support your knees, without locking (hyperextending) the joint. When learning straight-leg poses, such as Extended Triangle Pose (Utthita Trikonasana, Figure 8A), beginning students often ask me, *Should I lock my knees?* There is no simple answer to this question (although if there were, it would be no). Using asana therapeutically is nuanced, and calls upon you to develop body awareness. Take heart: With patience and practice, you can do this.

In straight-leg poses, the quadriceps muscles are engaged and active, lifting the kneecaps but without pushing them toward the backs of the joints. It is important to learn how to straighten the legs without locking them, using the quadriceps to create lift and support for the knee joints. This means that the quadriceps are firm in standing poses, and the kneecaps themselves are lifting toward the outer hips (rather than dropping toward the big toes). In order not to hyperextend while effecting this action, it is essential that the balls of the feet stay firmly weighted, rather than letting all the weight move toward the heels, and that the shins (lower legs) continue to move forward as the thighs (upper legs) are drawn up and back. We look at these actions in more detail in the asana sequence.

Your practice should serve you, not the other way around. Asana practice can be many different things to different people, and with yoga's contemporary popularity as a fitness activity, everywhere you look there seem to be posters and books with images of apparently perfect, young bodies demonstrating fantastical-looking poses. But an important guideline to follow when you are learning yoga is to listen to your *own* body. Do asana first and foremost for the benefits, both mental and physical: that means that you focus on the poses that make sense for your particular, individual needs. At some point, learning advanced asana may make sense, but for a beginning practitioner and someone who is doing therapeutic yoga, a basic, focused practice has the most to offer. Beware of the temptation to push yourself into a pose that your intuition or your body warns against, even if your teacher is urging you on and everyone else in the class seems to be doing it with ease. You can never know what others are feeling, but you do know what *you* are feeling in an asana, and listening to your inner wisdom will aid you greatly in your yoga practice.

Use props when you need them. B. K. S. Iyengar has made a significant contribution to using props in yoga, and it is one of the major elements that makes his system so therapeutic. Some common yoga props include blocks, straps, and blankets. They can be used in a variety of ways, such as supporting a part (or several parts) of the body in a pose, or extending your reach so that you can maintain correct alignment in a pose without straining, or simply bringing more attention to a body part or a physical action. The main use of props, however, is to adapt the poses to your needs, so that you can work in the poses at the level that is healthiest and safest for you. In the following section, "Poses for Healthy Knees," I suggest ways to use various props to create more comfort in different poses. Finding the most comfortable version of the pose for yourself is important: more comfort equals more relaxation in the pose, and more relaxation means fuller breath and, ultimately, more healing. As your strength and flexibility increase, you may find that you need fewer props to be comfortable in some poses, but there is no rush. More important is the quality of your experience in the pose at the moment. The props are intended to support and enhance that experience, so use them with enjoyment and in good health!

Finding a yoga teacher. If you are practicing yoga in a class, it is important that you work with a supportive, well-trained, safety-conscious teacher. If you have knee problems, your best bet is to study with a teacher who has an understanding of your condition. At the very least, choose someone who is sympathetic and encourages you to work gently and carefully. Your teacher should be able to help you adapt or find alternatives to such potentially knee-stressful poses as Lotus Pose (Padmasana) and Hero's Pose (Virasana, Figure 12A). And you should consider avoiding the more aggressive, acrobatic forms of yoga, such as Bikram Yoga, Ashtanga Yoga, and other strenuous forms of Vinyasa Yoga, at least until your knees are stabilized and pain-free. Keep in mind that your practice is meant to nurture you. I encourage you to adapt any pose or any sequence to better serve your needs. Caring for yourself through yoga practice is more important than mastering any particular pose.

ASANA

Staff Pose

DANDASANA

LENGTHENS THE HAMSTRINGS AND THE LIGAMENTS
BEHIND THE KNEES • BRINGS AWARENESS
▼ ▼ ▼ ▼ ▼ TO THE LEG MUSCLES

PROP: 1 nonskid mat

POSSIBLE PROPS: 1 blanket • 1 towel

Staff Pose (Dandasana, Figure 1A) is the basic seated posture, which you can practice to learn how to activate the quadriceps, energize the legs, and avoid bad habits, particularly hyperextension.

Sit on your mat and extend your legs in front of you, with your feet together and ankles flexed, so that your toes point directly upward. If you feel strain in your back or you experience restriction in the movement of the hip joints, place a folded blanket under your sitting bones (Figure 1B). This support will help with pelvic rotation and help you lengthen your spine with greater ease.

The torso should be at a right angle to the legs, with the crown of the head directly over the tailbone. Place the hands palms down and next to the hips. Rather than sinking onto the arms, lift away from them, lengthening through the spine, starting with the tailbone and lengthening up through the neck and head. Keep the shoulders relaxed and dropping away from the ears. If necessary, bend the elbows to bring ease to the shoulders.

The important work here is to learn to connect with the quadriceps muscles and activate them in a healthy manner. In physical therapy, an electrode device is often prescribed for just this purpose, but with practice your brain will do a perfectly adequate job of contacting underused muscles.

A common question is, *How do I know if my quadriceps are working?* In *30 Essential Yoga Poses*, yoga teacher and physical therapist Judith Lasater recommends this excellent method for connecting with these important support muscles. She says,

> . . . sit down on the floor, with the legs straight out in front and the quadriceps relaxed. . . . reach down with one hand and gently wiggle [your] kneecap from side to side. This should be easy to do and painless. . . . contract your quadriceps. This is easy to do if you imagine lifting [your] leg off the floor an inch . . . then try to move the kneecap from side to side. This is impossible if these muscles are contracting, because the quadriceps tendon presses the kneecap down into the leg and disallows any sideways movement of the kneecap.[1]

In other words, just the thought of contracting the quadriceps will send a signal to the muscles to activate them. This is a great method for learning how to

1. Judith Lasater, Ph.D., P.T., *30 Essential Yoga Poses: For Beginning Students and Their Teachers* (Berkeley, Calif.: Rodmell Press, 2003), 29.

work with the quadriceps in straight-leg poses. Underused muscles may not respond at first, but if you keep sending the message each time you practice, the nerve conduction will come alive and the quadriceps will begin to activate. With repetition over time, this action will strengthen the quadriceps, so they can do the job of supporting your knee joints.

When you are familiar with the work of the quads, sit in Staff Pose for a few moments, lengthening the legs from the hip sockets to the heels, and firming the quadriceps just above the inner knees. Rather than pushing the thighbones and shinbones toward the floor, draw the kneecaps gently toward the hips, as you continue to lengthen forward through the heels, so the backs of the legs lengthen forward and the fronts of the legs draw back in a countermovement.

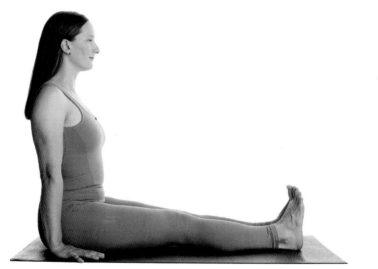

FIGURE 1A
STAFF POSE

The energy flow through the legs should be forward and back (hips sockets to feet), rather than up and down. If your heels come off the floor, you are hyperextending. See how long and active you can make the legs *without* the heels popping up. If the heels continue to pop up, then place a towel under the knees to protect them from hyperextending (Figure 1B). This support will let you know if you are pushing down on the knee joints.

Hold this pose for 30 seconds to 1 minute, bringing conscious awareness to the work of the legs. When you have learned how to bring about the dual energy of the legs in Staff Pose, you can apply these actions to working correctly in the standing poses.

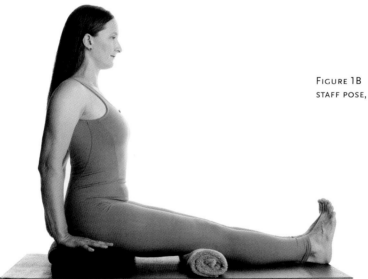

FIGURE 1B
STAFF POSE, WITH SUPPORT

Comfortable Seated Cross-Legged Pose

SUKHASANA

STRETCHES THE OUTER HIP MUSCLES
▼ ▼ ▼ ▼ ▼ INCREASES MOVEMENT IN THE HIP SOCKETS

PROPS: 1 nonskid mat • 1 blanket

POSSIBLE PROPS: 1 blanket • 1 washcloth

If you have knee problems, finding a comfortable sitting position can be challenging. This is especially true for meditators, who are often required to sit on the floor with little support. Although a lifetime of sitting in chairs is not good for the hips, knees, or spine, if your body is accustomed to a chair, the movements required to sit in a cross-legged meditation position may not be immediately available.

To practice Comfortable Seated Cross-Legged (Sukhasana, Figure 2), sit on your mat. Place a blanket under you for comfort, and fold your legs so that one ankle is crossed inside the other. *Dukha,* which means "suffering," is perhaps a better known Sanskrit word than *sukha,* which translates as "sweetness," meaning contentment, or even happiness. In this basic seated asana, the most common meditation posture, you are striving for the most comfortable position, one in which your body is content.

Notice if it is difficult to achieve movement at the hip sockets, or if the sacrum drops backward, causing the spine to slump. Notice also if the thighs are held so tightly in the hip sockets that the knees are lifted away from the floor, rather than dropping toward it. If any of these is the case, place a folded blanket under your sitting bones, which will help to lift and rotate the pelvis and make the posture more comfortable. This also tells you that tight outer hips, inner groins, or adductor muscles—or all three—may be contributing to tension in your knee joints. When movement at the larger joints is restricted, the smaller joints always have to compensate and, as discussed in the introduction, an especially tight area can pull joints out of alignment. If there is strain in the knees, placing a rolled washcloth behind one or both may help.

When you are as comfortable as possible, sit up tall, letting the thighbones relax as you lift from the hip sockets and the base of the spine. Find a comfortable place to rest your hands so that your arms and shoulders can relax without collapsing your spine, soften your eyes, and let your breath flow gently and naturally. Hold for at least 30 seconds and for as long as a few minutes, and then change the cross of your ankles and repeat on the other side. It is very important that you alternate sides. Be sure to hold the second, or nonhabitual, side at least as long as the side that comes more naturally, so that the hips are brought into more balance.

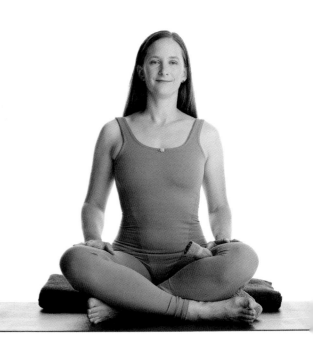

FIGURE 2
COMFORTABLE SEATED CROSS-LEGGED POSE

Cross-Legged Forward Bend Pose

SUKHASANA, VARIATION

INCREASES THE STRETCH OF OUTER HIP
ROTATORS • RELEASES TENSION IN THE GROINS, HIPS AND
▼ ▼ ▼ ▼ ▼ OUTER THIGHS • EASES LOWER BACK TENSION

PROPS: 1 nonskid mat • 1 blanket

POSSIBLE PROPS: 1 blanket • 1 block • 1 or 2 bolsters • 1 washcloth

Set up as for Comfortable Seated Cross-Legged Pose (Sukhasana, Figure 2). If you used a blanket under your sitting bones, you will need it for this variation. If you are less flexible, place a block in front of your ankles.

Keeping your sitting bones in contact with the blanket, reach forward into Cross-Legged Forward Bend Pose (Sukhasana, Variation, Figure 3). If you are working with a block, push it away from you with your fingertips, allowing your spine to follow as the block moves farther away as you come forward. Keep your neck relaxed, but don't worry about how close your head comes to the floor: instead, emphasize the forward movement and the length of the spine. In this way, both the hips and the back will receive maximum stretch, although you should feel it primarily in the outer hip rotators, including the gluteus muscles around the buttocks.

If your hips are tight, you may feel strain on the knees. Placing a bolster under each knee may help with this. *Do not bend forward if it hurts your knee to do so,* because the weight of your torso can take you farther into the stretch than your hips are ready for. And if the hips don't release, your knees will have to torque to allow this movement, particularly the inside knee, which is more compressed. A rolled washcloth, used as a spacer inside the knee joint, can be very effective for creating comfortable movement in this pose. As you cross your ankles, simply place the roll behind the inside knee, to lessen its compression. If this resolves the problem, in time you can practice without the roll and see how it feels, but be mindful and do use the roll as long as you need to in order to alleviate joint strain in this pose.

Once you have found maximum length in coming forward, you can relax onto your elbows or even let your head rest on the floor (or on the block) if that comes easily with no strain. Hold for 30 seconds to 1 minute. To come out, walk your hands along the floor back toward you, pushing up with your arms rather than pulling with your back. Change the cross of your ankles with the opposite ankle on top, and repeat on the other side.

FIGURE 3
CROSS-LEGGED FORWARD BEND POSE

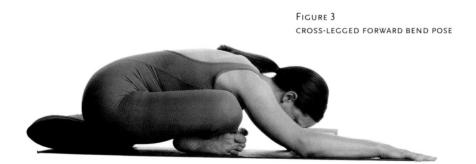

Half Downward-Facing Dog Pose

ARDHA ADHO MUKHA SVANASANA

STRETCHES THE HAMSTRINGS • FREES THE SPINE

▼ ▼ ▼ ▼ ▼ TEACHES HEALTHY MOVEMENT IN THE HIP SOCKETS

PROPS: 1 nonskid mat • a wall

To practice Half Downward-Facing Dog Pose (Ardha Adho Mukha Svanasana, Figure 4), position your mat perpendicular to a wall. Stand on the mat, facing the wall and a few inches from it. Have your feet parallel and hip-width apart. Note that for alignment purposes, "feet parallel" calls for toes pointing directly forward, and "hip-width" refers to the distance between the centers of the hip sockets—generally 4 to 6 inches—rather than the outer hips.

Place your hands on the wall, close into your body, just above your hips. Step back, letting your arms straighten and your chest drop but without letting your hands drop down the wall, until your spine is long and parallel to the floor. Keep your head in a neutral position, with your ears resting right between your arms. Lengthen your spine by stretching your tailbone away from the wall, creating maximum distance between your hands and your sitting bones, without letting your hands drop lower than the height of your hips. If your hamstrings are tight or the stretch feels too intense for any reason, you can modify it by keeping your hands a little higher on the wall and reducing the angle at your hip sockets.

Hold this pose for 30 seconds to 1 minute, breathing gently. It should be practiced often, and can be repeated several times in one practice session. Use this pose to practice the work of the quadriceps learned in Staff Pose (Dandasana, Figure 1A or Figure 1B), gently lifting through the fronts of the thighs without pushing the kneecaps backward.

FIGURE 4
HALF DOWNWARD-FACING DOG POSE

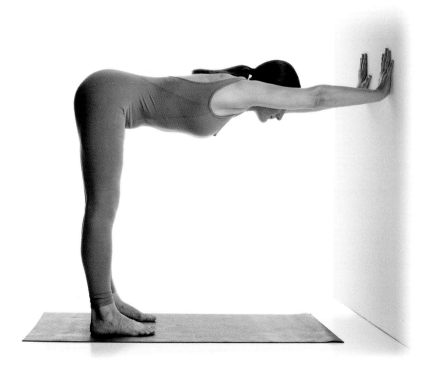

Seat-of-Power Pose

UTKATASANA

BUILDS STRENGTH IN THE MUSCLES OF THE
LEGS AND FEET • TEACHES HEALTHY ALIGNMENT
▼ ▼ ▼ ▼ ▼ STABILIZES THE KNEE AND ANKLE JOINTS

PROPS: 1 nonskid mat • a wall

POSSIBLE PROPS: 1 block • a mirror or a friend

For this version of Seat-of-Power Pose (Utkatasana, Figure 5), stand with your mat perpendicular to the wall, your back against the wall, and your feet parallel and hip-width apart. On an exhalation, walk your feet forward, sliding your back down the wall, until your legs form right angles, with your knees directly over your heels.

Attention to correct alignment is very important in this pose! The feet should be parallel, which means that the outer edges of the feet should be parallel to the edges of the mat. This may feel overly turned in, because the balls of the feet are wider than the heels. The heels must turn slightly away from each other to bring the feet into a parallel position. Or look at the line between the big toe and the second toe on each foot: these lines should also be parallel and may be easier to see. Your knees should stay firmly over the heels and not knock in toward each other or splay outward. The arches should be lifted and ankles balanced, which means that the inner and outer anklebones should be, as closely as possible, the same distance from the floor, so that the greatest energy of the arch is under the center of the foot rather than off to one side.

Although this is a lot to think about, it is attention to detail in this pose that provides maximum benefit, strengthening the knee joint as a whole, rather

FIGURE 5
SEAT-OF-POWER POSE

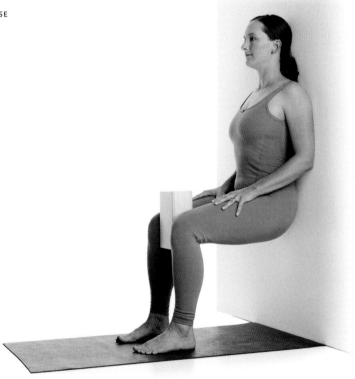

than reinforcing existing patterns. To keep the legs steady and conscious, it can be helpful to hold a block between the knees. And to understand the tendencies of the feet, it can be very helpful to work with lifting the toes. Try to lift all ten toes equally, pressing through the four corners of the feet and keeping the ankles balanced. (Notice and try to adjust if your ankles and arches sink to the inside or outside. Using a mirror or having a friend look at your feet once or twice as you learn this pose can give you helpful information for your practice.) Keep the arches and the ankles balanced and energized as you replace your toes lightly onto the floor, keeping them spread and keeping the weight in the four corners.

Hold this pose for 30 seconds, and gradually build up to 1 minute, or even, eventually, 2 minutes, to strengthen the knees. Breathe gently and keep your awareness focused on your alignment while you are in the pose. To come out, press through your feet and slide your sitting bones back up the wall. Rest with your sitting bones against the wall, and then repeat the pose a second time.

If the pose feels too difficult at the beginning, keep your hips a bit higher on the wall, rather than coming all the way to 90 degrees, working with your alignment and your breath, and work toward the 90-degree position as you get stronger. If 30 seconds is too long, start with 15 or 20 seconds. You will feel a strong sensation in your quads as they become tired, so come out when you need to; with practice, you will increase your time.

Tree Pose

VRKSASANA

STRENGTHENS THE MUSCLES OF THE FEET,
ANKLES, KNEES, AND LEGS • STRETCHES THE
INNER THIGH MUSCLES • TEACHES THE THIGH
▼ ▼ ▼ ▼ ▼ TO ROTATE IN THE HIP SOCKET

PROP: 1 nonskid mat

POSSIBLE PROP: a wall

Begin Tree Pose (Vrksasana, Figure 6) by standing on your mat with the feet together, and
aligning your shoulders over your hips and the
crown of your head over the tailbone. Press
down firmly through the four corners of your
feet, lengthen your tailbone toward the floor,
and feel the rest of the spine lifting from the
tailbone, lengthening upward. Gently focus
your eyes at eye level, with your jawline parallel to the floor.

On an exhalation, shift your weight onto

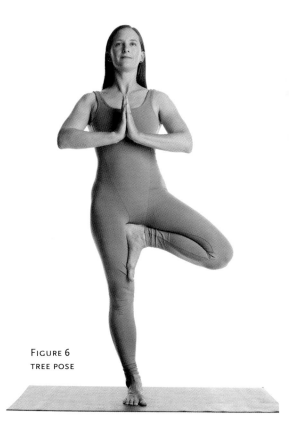

FIGURE 6
TREE POSE

your right leg, keeping your eyes level and focused as you move. Inhale, lift your left foot off the floor, and take hold of your left ankle with your left hand, drawing your foot toward your groin. As you place the sole of your left foot against your inner right thigh, press firmly down through your right foot to help yourself balance. Once the foot is in place, make sure that you are not using it to push yourself to the right: instead, firm the inner thigh muscles of the right leg against the sole of the foot, to help you stay centered and to keep the foot from slipping. Staying focused on the midline of your body, let go of your ankle, and bring your hands to *Namaste,* or Prayer Position, by gently pressing your palms together in front of your chest.

While in Tree Pose, keep your shoulders relaxed and your spine long, lifting from the strength of the standing leg. The eyes stay softly focused, the abdomen is gently engaged, the sacrum moves into the body, and the left foot and the inner right thigh continue to press together. One of the challenges is remembering to do all these things at once: this becomes much easier with practice.

If you find it difficult to stay balanced, learn the pose standing near a wall, so that you can practice with one hand placed on the wall as you become accustomed to standing on one leg. Once balance becomes easier, you can lift the arms overhead, palms facing each other, for more stretch of the spine and a more challenging experience of balance.

Balancing on one leg is very strengthening for the knee and ankle joints, but may be quite difficult at first, especially if those joints are misaligned. Remember to breathe while practicing this pose. Have faith that ease will come with consistent practice!

Challenging Balance: Eyes Closed

STRENGTHENS THE MUSCLES OF THE FEET, ANKLES,
KNEES, AND LEGS • BRINGS KNEES AND ANKLES INTO
ALIGNMENT • PREVENTS ATROPHY OF THE KNEE MUSCLES
▼ ▼ ▼ ▼ ▼ IMPROVES MENTAL FOCUS AND BALANCE SKILLS

PROP: 1 nonskid mat

Challenging Balance: Eyes Closed (Figure 7) is very popular with physical therapists and alternative health care practitioners. I learned it from Encinitas, California, chiropractor Bill Lerner and have found it to yield amazing results.[2] Although it can be challenging to learn, there is no downside, and it is very beneficial to keep working on it. Without the orientation of your eyes to assist you, your feet, ankles, and knees have to find much truer alignment to keep you balanced. This strengthens and stabilizes the joints, and it helps to prevent atrophy in muscles that would otherwise be underused.

2. Bill Lerner, D.C., personal communication with the author, August 2002.

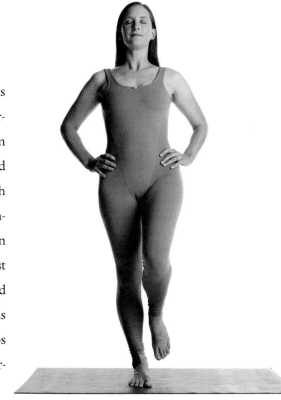

FIGURE 7
CHALLENGING BALANCE: EYES CLOSED

Stand on your mat with your feet together. Focus your eyes and press down through your feet. Place your hands on your hips, or if balance is very difficult, stretch your arms out to your sides in a T position. As you shift your weight to one foot, both feel and visualize the line of the spine stretching upward, so that you are energetically connected to the floor through the four corners of one foot, and to the ceiling through the crown of the head. Once groundedness, length, and center are established, lift the other foot a few inches off the floor, find your balance, and, staying focused, close your eyes. You will experience your standing foot and ankle flickering; try to balance the inner and outer ankle as evenly as possible, establishing stability. Breathe calmly and gently. Try to stay balanced for 10 slow breaths, and then place your foot back on the floor, open your eyes, and repeat the process on the other side.

Initially, 10 breaths (or even 5) may feel impossible. In this case, start with 3 and gradually increase them as your ability to balance improves. With practice, you will feel your knee joint strengthen and alignment improve. Often you will be able to feel this happen as you balance, which is very motivating! This important exercise should be practiced daily or even several times a day, and can be done anywhere that you have a few quiet moments to concentrate. When it is part of your yoga practice, stand on your mat. However, the bare floor will do when you are in your kitchen waiting for your kettle to boil or your toast to pop!

Extended Triangle Pose

UTTHITA TRIKONASANA

STRETCHES THE HAMSTRINGS, CALVES, AND INNER THIGHS

ENGAGES AND STRENGTHENS THE QUADRICEPS

▼ ▼ ▼ ▼ ▼ IMPROVES MOBILITY OF THE HIP SOCKETS

PROPS: 1 nonskid mat • 1 block

POSSIBLE PROP: a wall

Stand on your mat with your feet approximately 4 feet apart (or a bit farther apart if you are tall). The distance between your feet should be roughly the length of one of your own legs, so that the triangle shape your legs make with the floor is equilateral. If this feels unstable, or if it feels that the hamstrings or the groins are overstretching, place the feet slightly closer to each other until the pose is more comfortable. Place a block next to your outer right ankle.

Turn your right foot out 90 degrees, so that your toes point directly toward the end of your mat, and turn your left foot in about halfway, so that your toes turn in about 45 degrees toward your right foot. Press firmly and equally into both feet for balance, and as you press down through the feet, gently engage the quadriceps, so that the front thighs are firm and lifted. Inhale, and lift the arms so that they are parallel with the floor, taking care to keep the tops of the shoulders relaxed as you stretch the fingertips away from one another.

Before coming into Extended Triangle Pose (Utthita Trikonasana, Figure 8A), focus on several actions: First, press into the outer edge of the left (back) foot and into the ball of the right (front) foot. Keeping the quadriceps firm, externally rotate the front thigh, turning the inner thigh gently outward. Finally, keeping the front thigh turned out, rotate the spine away from the front leg, so that the navel turns up toward the left arm. With all of this in mind, you are ready to move into Extended Triangle Pose.

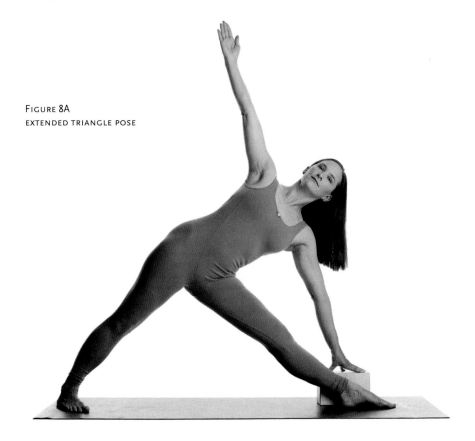

FIGURE 8A
EXTENDED TRIANGLE POSE

Dropping the right thighbone in the hip socket, feel the pelvis swinging up to the left, and let the torso stretch to the right, leaning over the front leg. Keep the spine as long as possible, lengthening from the tailbone to the crown of the head, and bring the right hand to the block, stretching between the fingertips of each hand as the left hand extends straight up toward the ceiling. The hand on the block will help you balance, but should not take your weight, which stays firmly—and as equally as possible—in the legs.

Hold this pose for 30 seconds to 1 minute, breathing gently. While in Extended Triangle Pose, focus on the actions you established before coming into the pose: Press into the outer heel of the back foot, and widen and firm the ball of the front foot; keep the quadriceps firm and lifted as you gently externally rotate the front thigh; and keep the spine and arms long and energized as you turn the navel away from the floor and toward the top hand.

The work of the feet and quads is important in order to prevent hyperextension of the front knee. The knees should not bend: if they do, the quads cannot engage, and strengthening the thigh muscles is a key benefit of this pose. Nor should the knee be locked: this pose is an opportunity to work on finding a neutral, rather than hyperextended, straight position for the knee joint. For those with acute hyperextension, this neutral position often feels as if the knee were bent. You can test whether your quadriceps are working by placing your hand on your knee to see if it is stable, as you learned to do in Staff Pose (Figure 1A or Figure 1B). The kneecap should not wiggle, and the muscles just above it should be firm. (When in Extended Triangle Pose, it is safer to do the knee test with your back heel pressing against the wall, for stability.) In what I call the "neutral straight position," the shin presses slightly forward, as if the leg were about to bend, while the thigh is drawn back and up, resisting the bending action.

Sometimes there is an intense stretch on the ligaments of the inner knee when a student first learns this pose. Working with the quadriceps and learning to find the neutral straight position, rather than locking the joint, should both help. However, if those ligaments feel as if they are overstretching, do the pose with the front foot placed 2 to 3 feet from the wall, and come just halfway

FIGURE 8B
EXTENDED TRIANGLE POSE, WITH WALL SUPPORT

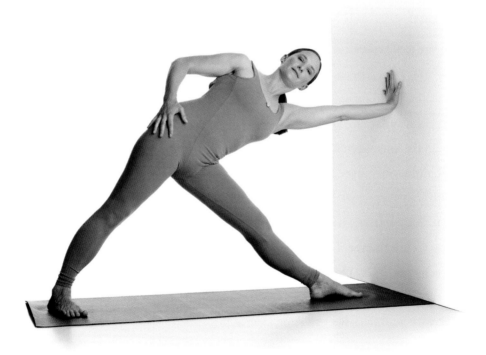

down (Figure 8B). Let the fingertips rest on the wall for support at the level of the spine, rather than bringing the hand all the way down to the block. You can use this variation until you feel ready for the full pose.

To come out, bend the front knee slightly, pushing off the front foot while reaching with the top arm to bring the spine upright. Ground your feet for balance, take a breath, and then carefully turn your feet through center and then to the left, repeating the entire process on the second side.

Warrior II Pose

VIRABHADRASANA II

STRENGTHENS THE MUSCLES OF THE FEET
AND KNEES • STABILIZES THE KNEE AND ANKLE JOINTS
▼ ▼ ▼ ▼ ▼ OPENS THE INNER THIGHS AND HIPS

PROP: 1 nonskid mat

Stand on your mat with your feet placed as in Extended Triangle Pose (Figure 8A): 4 to 4½ feet apart, front foot turned all the way out, and back foot turned halfway in. Keeping your shoulders relaxed, on an inhalation, raise your arms so that they are parallel with the floor. The arms are long, with the hands stretching through the fingertips and away from each other, and the spine lengthening through the center of the body.

Keep the back leg strong and grounded, and bend the front knee. As you move farther into the pose, resist the impulse to drop your torso toward the bending leg. Instead, stay focused on stretching the arms evenly away from each other and on stretching the spine up. The strong back leg will help with this, and it is useful to imagine that leg resisting, as if it were trying to pull you back up to standing, while the front thigh moves toward the floor.

When the front leg is bent to a 90-degree angle and the spine is still centered, you are in Warrior II Pose (Virabhadrasana II, Figure 9). Make sure that your front knee is aligned directly over your heel and ankle. It is common for the knee to drop toward the inner arch of the foot, but this is detrimental to the knee joint; correct alignment, on the other hand, is highly therapeutic. This means that concentration is essential for maximum benefit from this pose. If your hips are tight and you aren't able to keep your front knee aligned, don't bend the knee as deeply: alignment is more important than how far you fold into any pose. This is especially true when you are working for therapeutic benefit.

Hold the pose for 30 seconds to 1 minute. As you breathe in the pose, gently rotate the spine away from the front leg, which stretches the hips. You will

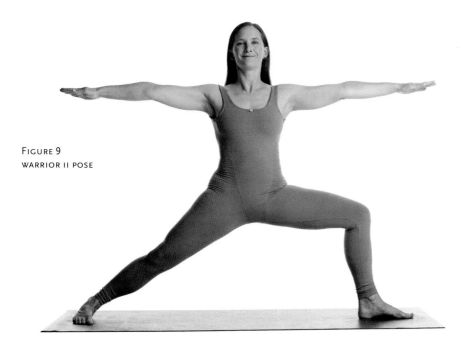

FIGURE 9
WARRIOR II POSE

feel your knee wanting to drop inward as you do this, but resist and keep your knee very steady. Keep the tops of your shoulders soft and relaxed as the spine and arms continue to lengthen.

In any standing pose, you can work with balancing and strengthening the feet and ankles, lifting the toes as you did in Seat-of-Power Pose (Figure 5). Warrior II Pose is an excellent asana in which to bring your attention to your feet, and work on strengthening and aligning your arches and anklebones. As you challenge yourself to hold this pose for a longer time, you will feel your legs getting stronger, but you will also know when you are at your limit. When it is time to come out of the pose, simply straighten the front leg and lift out of it. Once your leg is straight, carefully turn the feet and repeat the pose on the second side.

Warrior I Pose

VIRABHADRASANA I

STRENGTHENS THE MUSCLES OF THE FEET AND
KNEES • STABILIZES THE KNEE AND ANKLE JOINTS
▼ ▼ ▼ ▼ ▼ STRETCHES THE HIP FLEXORS AND CALF MUSCLES

PROP: 1 nonskid mat

To practice Warrior I Pose (Virabhadrasana I, Figure 10), stand on your mat, with your feet 4 to 4½ feet apart. Turn your right foot all the way out. You will be turning your torso away from your back leg, so turn your left foot in farther than in the previous poses, at least 45 degrees and up to 60 degrees if you can do so comfortably. It is important that your back foot turn in adequately, so as not to strain the knee when you turn the pelvis away from it.

Place your hands on your hips and, pressing your feet firmly into the floor, turn your hips toward your front leg, bringing your hips as close to level, or square, as possible, without straining. Center your spine on the midline between your two legs, facing the right end of your mat. As you lengthen the spine by lifting from the floor of the pelvis, press into the outer edge of the back foot, keeping the arch active and the inner left thigh muscles firm and lifted. Continue to lengthen upward through the spine, and keep the chest lifted and open.

While you are learning the pose, the hands can remain on the hips for stability. As you get more comfortable holding Warrior I Pose, you can stretch the arms overhead and reach through the fingertips. The arms are placed next to the ears and the palms turn toward each other. Adding the overhead arm stretch does not appreciably affect the primary benefits for the knees, but does give a nice stretch to the shoulders, chest, and upper spine, which is energizing and feels great. In either version, keep the shoulders relaxed. When you feel ready, lift the toes of both feet. This action stabilizes the ankles and the knees even more by strengthening the muscles around them, giving added focus to correcting the alignment of these joints.

Hold Warrior I Pose for 30 seconds to 1 minute, or longer if you are strong enough to do so without strain. To exit, simply straighten the front leg and lift up, keeping the feet grounded and bringing the arms down if they are lifted. Once the front leg is completely straight, carefully turn the feet through center and then to the other side to repeat the pose to the left.

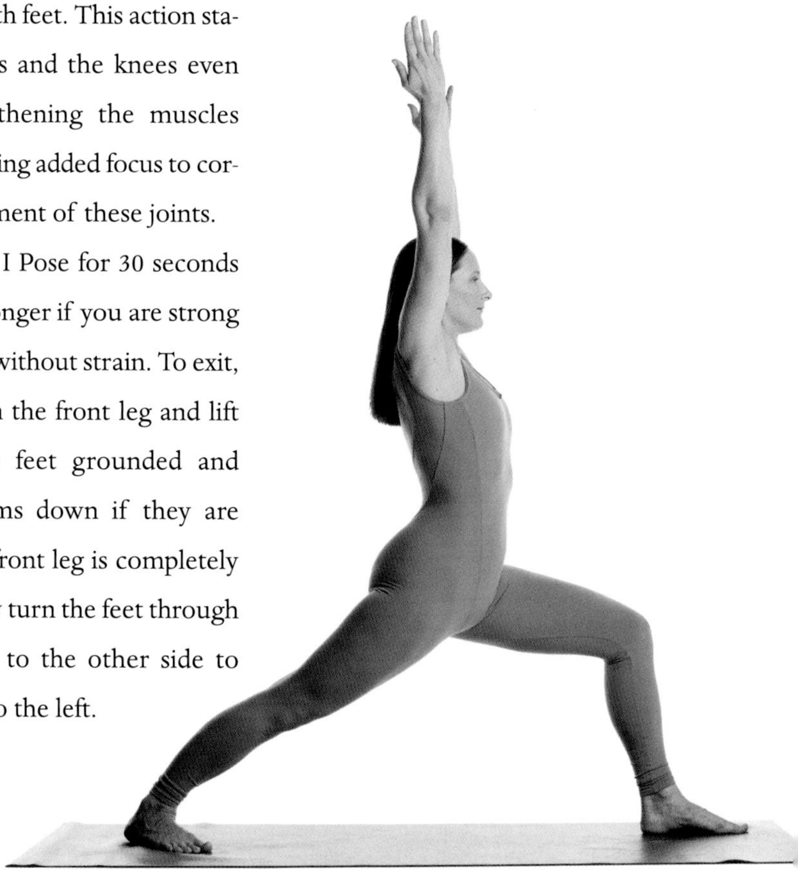

FIGURE 10
WARRIOR I POSE

Half-Frog Pose

ARDHA BHEKASANA

▼ ▼ ▼ ▼ ▼ STRETCHES THE QUADRICEPS AND HIP FLEXORS

PROPS: 1 nonskid mat • 1 blanket

POSSIBLE PROP: 1 strap

The quadriceps, which are the muscles of the front thigh, are very strong, dense, and active muscles. The psoas, which are the core support muscles that wrap around from the inner thighs around the front of the pelvis to connect to the lower back, tighten every time you take a step and every time you sit down. So it is common for these muscles to be tight. The quadriceps attach directly to the knee joints, so tight quads can pull on the patella and cause strain. Another concern is imbalance. The typical pattern of strong, tight outer quads is stressful for the knee joints and also affects the gait in walking and running. A gait that is misaligned adds to knee strain.

Keeping the quadriceps and iliopsoas stretched and supple is essential for healthy knees, and is especially important for athletes, who often have to overuse these muscles.

There are many possible quadriceps and psoas stretches to choose from in yoga. Half-Frog Pose (Ardha Bhekasana, Figure 11) is a good basic one to start with. To begin, place a folded blanket on your mat. Lie face down, resting your forehead on your left arm. Bend your right knee, bringing your foot toward your right hip, and reach back with your right hand to take hold of your foot. If reaching is difficult, loop a strap around your foot or ankle. Keep the weight centered, with the sacrum grounded toward the belly and both front hipbones pressing gently and evenly into the floor. Draw the foot gently toward the outer hip, lengthening the front of the thigh back toward the knee as the foot comes toward you.

Breathe comfortably and hold for 30 seconds to 1 minute. You should feel the stretch primarily along the front of the right hip and thigh, and there should be no feeling of strain in the knee. If you feel discomfort in the knee, back off as needed or release altogether: never force any pose. To come out, let go of the foot and bring it back to the floor. Repeat on the other side.

FIGURE 11
HALF-FROG POSE

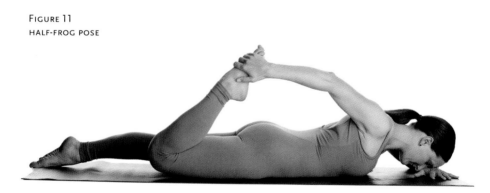

Hero's Pose

VIRASANA

RELEASES THE FRONT THIGHS AND DEEP HIP FLEXORS
ROTATES THE THIGHS INTERNALLY AND INCREASES MOBILITY OF THE HIP
SOCKETS • STRETCHES THE SHINS, ANKLES, AND FEET • STRENGTHENS
▼ ▼ ▼ ▼ ▼ THE MUSCLES OF THE ARCHES THAT SUPPORT THE FEET

PROPS: 1 nonskid mat • 1 block • 1 blanket

POSSIBLE PROPS: 1 bolster • 2 washcloths or 2 small towels

A word of caution about Hero's Pose: This pose is not for everyone, and can be tricky for those with knee problems. However, it offers benefits that make it worthwhile for those who can work with it safely. So approach Hero's Pose (Virasana, Figure 12A) cautiously. It is essential that you prop yourself up to the appropriate height, so that you experience absolutely no knee pain in the pose. Although when first learning Hero's Pose, you may feel a mild stretch in the tendons that stretch over the knees, the key word is "mild." If you have anterior cruciate ligament (ACL) injuries, you should sit high enough that there is *no* stretching sensation in the fronts of the knees (Figure 12B). For maximum benefit, sit in Hero's Pose for 3 to 5 minutes, long enough for the groins and quadriceps to relax into the pose. When you are preparing for the pose, remember that any sensation you feel in your knees will increase exponentially in a short amount of time, and set up your props accordingly.

The props needed for this pose are especially individual. Make sure that you practice on a comfortable surface. You can place a blanket on top of your mat so that your shinbones have a soft surface to rest on. You will be sitting with your sitting bones between your feet: having both a block and a folded blanket to work with will give you the flexibility to adjust the height of your props. A block by itself will work for many students, but if your quadriceps or shins (or both) are tight, add more height by placing a folded blanket on top of the block.

FIGURE 12A
HERO'S POSE

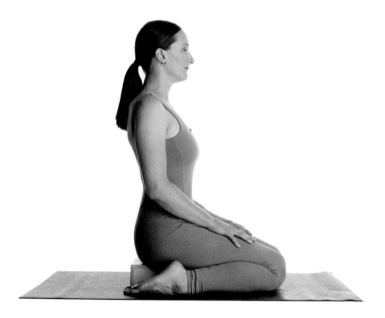

If you need even more height, use a bolster. If you are looser in the quads and the groins, use just the blanket. Adapt the props to your own requirements, always adjusting for complete ease and comfort.

Come to your hands and knees on your blanket, placing your block or blanket (or both) between your feet. If you are using a block, place it in the wide position between the feet, so that your feet come just outside the hips rather than under them. Sit back onto your supporting props, and take a moment to check in with how your knees feel. Once you are comfortable in the pose, look for three important elements.

FIGURE 12B
HERO'S POSE, WITH SUPPORT

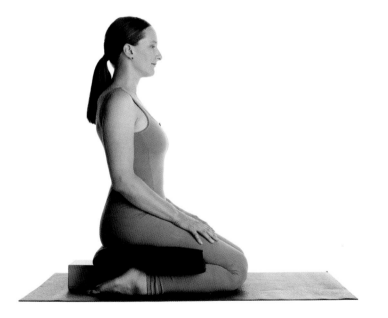

First, your feet should be positioned with the toes pointing directly back, rather than in toward each other, and keep the inner ankles long. It's fine if you have mild sensation in the shins or in the arches of the feet, because you want these areas to stretch. However, if your shins or feet are very tight, the stretch may be too intense. In this case, placing a rolled or folded washcloth or small towel under the front of each ankle can help reduce the sensation of the stretch and make the pose more comfortable. Often students are not sure how much is too much. You are your own best judge of how much sensation your body and mind can tolerate. Remember that pain should be avoided. Overly intense sensation, which is sensation that captures your attention so completely that your body, mind, and breath cannot relax in the pose, crosses the line into pain. If this is the case, definitely use props to create more comfort.

Next, in the classic pose, the knees touch, which is fine if it is comfortable. But this position does not work for everyone and should not be forced. Don't allow the knees to slide out wider than the hips, and place them so that they point toward, rather than away from, each other. Bring them toward each other, but don't go farther than is comfortable for you.

Finally, don't slump! Sit up tall, lifting from the hip sockets and supporting the spine at the sacrum. Lengthen your spine with your shoulders placed directly over your pelvis and the crown of your head in line with your tailbone. If your sacrum drops back, or you can't get any movement at the hip sockets, you will strain your back trying to lengthen your spine. Increase the height of your props to create more movement of the pelvis and more ease and freedom in the spine.

Practice for 1 minute, breathing gently, to start with, and increase your time as you feel ready. Eventually, you can sit for 5 minutes or more, as long as there is no knee strain and as long as you can maintain the length and energy of your spine. As you sit for longer periods, an added benefit of the pose is increased back strength. While you sit, spend some time breathing quietly. Close your eyes and focus on your experience. Staying present and mindful will help ensure that you don't overdo the pose.

Sometimes this position can restrict circulation to the lower legs. As your muscles loosen up with practice, circulation will move more easily through the pose. In the meantime, if your knees or feet fall asleep, it is time to come out.

When you are ready, use your hands on the floor to lift yourself carefully back onto your hands and knees. Gently move your props out of the way. Bring your feet toward each other until your big toes touch, and slide your knees away from each other until they are a bit wider than the hips. Then drop your hips down toward your heels, and rest your forehead on your mat, or, if it is more comfortable, fold your arms and rest your head on your forearms. This position is called Child's Pose (Balasana), and is a counterpose for the knees.

It is common for beginners to have some tingling in the knees after Hero's Pose: this is fine if it isn't extreme. Rest in Child's Pose until your knees feel neutral and your back is relaxed. Then use your hands to push yourself up to kneeling and then stand up. If you don't feel ready to stand, sit in Staff Pose (Figure 1A or Figure 1B) until you do.

Downward-Facing Dog Pose

AHDO MUKHA SVANASANA

STRENGTHENS THE LEGS • CREATES MOBILITY
OF THE HIP SOCKETS • STRETCHES THE HAMSTRINGS AND THE
▼ ▼ ▼ ▼ ▼ CALVES • OPENS AND ENERGIZES THE WHOLE BODY

PROP: 1 nonskid mat

Come onto your hands and knees on your mat. Draw your sitting bones back toward your heels while stretching your arms out in front of you, with your hands on the floor, placed shoulder-width apart. Keeping your arms long and straight, and your hands grounded in front of your shoulders, tuck your toes under. On an inhalation, lift your knees off the floor, straightening your legs and lifting your hips up and back.

Hold Downward-Facing Dog Pose (Adho Mukha Svanasana, Figure 13) for 30 seconds to 1 minute, breathing gently. Your feet should be hip-width apart and parallel with one another. Let your head rest in neutral between the arms, with your neck relaxed. While in "Down Dog," press into your hands and lengthen your spine, lifting through your sitting bones; simultaneously, stretch downward through the legs, allowing the heels to move closer to the floor. Keep your legs straight, with the quadriceps muscles firm and lifted, and the thigh-bones drawing back against the hamstrings; and gently activate the abdominal muscles, lifting into the body so that the belly feels concave.

To come out, come back to your hands and knees on an exhalation. Repeat this pose several times if you like, resting in Child's Pose (see the description on page 63) briefly between repetitions.

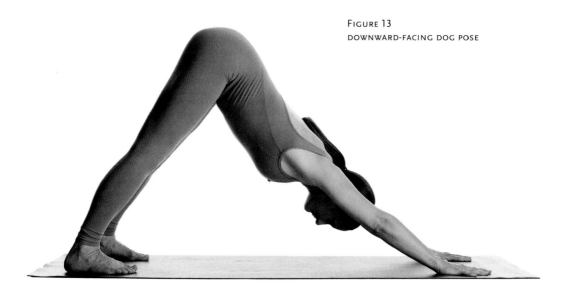

FIGURE 13
DOWNWARD-FACING DOG POSE

Thread the Needle I

PROPS: 1 nonskid mat • 1 blanket

POSSIBLE PROP: 1 strap

Flexibility of the outer hips is essential for healthy knees, because tight hips pull strongly on the kneecaps while restricting range of motion in the hip sockets. Various outer hip stretches release the hip rotator muscles. I present two beginning-level stretches in this book: Thread the Needle I and Thread the Needle II (the latter follows on page 68).

To practice Thread the Needle I (Figure 14), place a folded blanket on your mat. Lie on your back, with your knees bent and with your feet flat on the floor and hip-width apart. Keeping your left foot in place, cross your right ankle over your left thigh, resting it just above your left knee. The right ankle is firmly flexed, with the inner ankle open; the toes point toward the ceiling; and the heel moves away from the ankle. Lift the left foot off the floor, and draw the left thigh toward the chest, keeping the left knee bent. Reach around with both hands, threading the right hand through the space between the legs, and clasp the back of the left thigh. (Often this stretch is taught holding the shin, but this can compress the knee: holding behind the thigh is a safer approach.) If reaching is difficult, wrap a strap around the back of the thigh and hold one end in each hand. Keep the right ankle flexed, and bring the left thigh toward the chest until you feel the stretch in the outer right hip.

Hold this stretch for 30 seconds to 1 minute. Breathe and feel the hip muscles soften and release their tight grip on the outer pelvis. For a deeper stretch, use a little pressure of the right elbow on the inner right thigh to press the rotating leg away from yourself as you bring the leg you are clasping toward yourself. Make sure to press on the leg nearer to the top of the thigh than to the knee. This oppositional movement increases the distance those muscles need to lengthen and increases the intensity of the stretch. Move slowly and don't work beyond your comfort level.

To come out, release your leg (or the strap), and bring your left foot back to the floor before uncrossing your right leg. With both feet on the floor, cross the other way—left ankle over right thigh—to repeat on the opposite side.

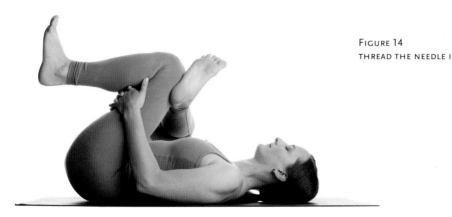

FIGURE 14
THREAD THE NEEDLE I

Thread the Needle II

PROPS: 1 nonskid mat • a chair

Once you are comfortable doing the reclining version of this stretch (Thread the Needle I, Figure 14), try Thread the Needle II (Figure 15A and Figure 15B). Although in this variation you do not actually thread your arm, you do place your legs in the same configuration and it works the same muscle group.

In this variation, the stretch moves deeper into the outer hip, because the seated position adds gravitational pull, allowing the spine to hang from the pelvis. This pulls on the hip muscles, and is a pleasant release for the spine and back muscles. Another benefit of Thread the Needle II is that you can do it anywhere there is an available chair. Well, almost anywhere. Unfortunately there is not quite enough room on an airplane for this exercise, at least not in coach!

To begin, place a chair on your mat. Sit at the front edge of the chair seat. Place your feet firmly on the floor; make sure that your feet are parallel and hip-width apart. Sit up tall, lifting out of the hip sockets and bringing the sacrum gently in and up. Then cross the right ankle over the left thigh, resting it in a flexed position just above the left knee. Place your hands on your hips and, keeping the front of your spine very long and your right foot flexed, begin to lean forward (Figure 15A). Your head should be in a neutral position, continuing the line of the spine, rather than dropping or lifting from the shoulders. Soften your neck and your face. Keeping the right foot flexed, allow your right thigh to relax, dropping into the pull of gravity. But don't push it downward: simply let the thighbone relax in the hip socket and let gravity do the work as you continue to lengthen forward from the hip sockets. You should feel the stretch deep in your right hip. Breathe gently and feel your muscles releasing.

This first stage of the pose may be intense: if so, that is enough for the time being. Don't go to the next level until the first stage is comfortable. When that is the case, allow your arms to relax toward the floor, in front of your right shin. Then drop your head and relax your spine (Figure 15B). Make sure that you have lengthened forward to the maximum that is comfortable before you release downward: the forward movement is the most important. As you release the spine, you add more

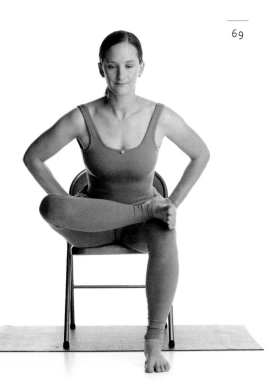

FIGURE 15A
THREAD THE NEEDLE II, STAGE ONE

weight to the hip stretch and you feel the sensation increase. Stay at an intensity level that feels reasonable to you. Your mind may be talking to you about the sensations that you feel in the hips, but neither the mind nor the hip rotators should be screaming or burning. If they are, go back to the first stage or practice Thread the Needle I (Figure 14). These are dense muscles, so progress will be gradual.

Hold the pose for 30 seconds to 1 minute, working up to 2 minutes as your comfort level allows. As the outer hip muscles release, movement in the hip sockets becomes freer and more efficient, which reduces strain on the knees.

To come out, keep the head relaxed as you bring the hands back to the hips. Press into the left foot and lengthen the spine forward to come up, leading with the sternum. Once your spine is upright, place your right hand under your right knee and lift it away from the floor. As the knee comes up, it is safe and easy to uncross the leg and place the right foot on the floor. Then you will be ready to do the other side.

FIGURE 15B
THREAD THE NEEDLE II, STAGE TWO

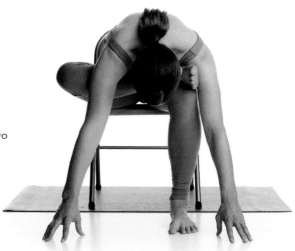

Reclining Twist Pose

JATARA PARIVARTANASANA

RELEASES THE SPINE, SHOULDERS, AND OUTER HIPS

▼ ▼ ▼ ▼ ▼ STRETCHES THE PSOAS AND ILIOTIBIAL BAND

PROPS: 1 nonskid mat • 1 blanket

To practice Reclining Twist Pose (Jatara Parivartanasana, Figure 16), lie on your mat with a folded blanket under your back for comfort. Bend your knees, place your feet flat on the floor, and stretch your arms out to your sides in a T, palms up. Cross the right knee over the left, letting the right foot hang over to the left side, so that the right knee is directly on top of the left knee. Scoot your hips slightly to the right, and then drop both knees to the left, coming onto your left side. Keep your head neutral, with your nose pointed toward the ceiling and your neck relaxed. (Scooting your hips in the opposite direction of your knees, so that your spine is at a slight diagonal before you twist, allows the spine to move more freely, so make sure to do this movement before moving fully into the pose.)

Allow the legs to relax, providing an anchor for the pose, and let the belly stretch from the left hip toward the right shoulder. Relax the right shoulder and let the right arm feel heavy. Breathe gently for 30 seconds to 1 minute. To come out, lift your knees and bring your pelvis under you again, centering your spine. Cross your legs with your left knee on top, and repeat to the other side.

The primary benefits of Reclining Twist Pose are to neutralize the spine and release the back muscles at the end of a practice session; the twist itself provides a counterpose to the previous poses, rather than directly benefiting the knees. This cross-legged version, however, does have a direct benefit for the knees: it is one of the few stretches that helps to release the iliotibial (IT) band, the thick rope of tissue that runs down along the outer thigh.

Caution: If you have sacroiliac problems, do not practice this version of the pose. Instead, do a simpler version, with both knees bent but not crossed.

FIGURE 16
RECLINING TWIST POSE

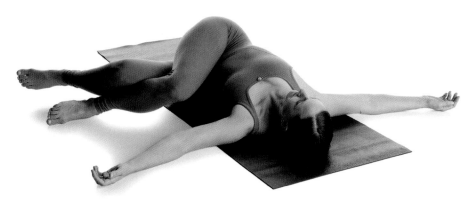

Relaxation Pose

SAVASANA

AIDS THE BODY'S HEALING AND REPAIR FUNCTIONS
KEEPS THE NERVOUS SYSTEM HEALTHY
▼ ▼ ▼ ▼ ▼ SUPPORTS OPTIMUM HEALTH

PROPS: 1 nonskid mat • 1 blanket • 1 bolster • a timer

POSSIBLE PROPS: 1 blanket or 1 bath towel • 1 washcloth

Students are often tempted to skip Relaxation Pose (Savasana, Figure 17), but it is an essential part of yoga practice. During the relaxation phase of practice, the body and mind integrate the work that you have done, the muscles relax, and the nervous system unwinds. Although it may not seem that these benefits directly affect the knees, regular relaxation is important to the body's ability to heal itself. If the body and mind are constantly active, the nervous system is always in overdrive, taking energy from maintenance and repair functions. It is only when your nervous system is allowed to take regular time off that these systems can operate optimally. Because of this, Relaxation Pose is a key element of any therapeutic practice. It benefits the whole system: body, mind, and spirit. This is what is meant by holistic health.

Position your mat and place a folded blanket on top of it. Lie down on the blanket. Take the time to create comfort for yourself. Treat yourself to a bolster under your knees, so that they can relax completely. Options to make Relaxation Pose even more delicious include a folded blanket (or a bath towel) under the head and neck and a washcloth over the eyes. Position them now.

Stretch your arms out to your sides, palms turned up, and let them relax. Let your knees relax away from each other; let your feet relax away from each other. Relax completely, letting your breath find its natural rhythm and letting your mind clear.

Stay in Relaxation Pose for 5 to 10 minutes: stay longer if you have the time and inclination. Setting a timer will free your mind from worry about falling asleep.

When you are ready to come out, take your time and move gently. Moving consciously with your breath, bend your knees, one by one, bringing your feet onto the bolster. With an exhalation, roll onto one side. (Your eye cover will slip off by itself.) Keep your eyes closed, so that they can adjust slowly to the light.

Stay resting on your side for a few breaths. When you are ready, use the support of your arms to bring yourself up to a sitting position and back into the world of activity.

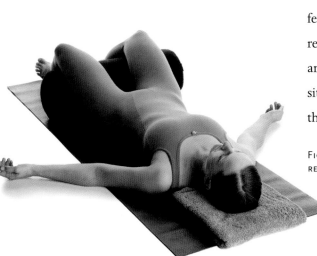

FIGURE 17
RELAXATION POSE

Putting the Poses Together

Many people find that making the time for practice is the biggest obstacle. For this reason, I have designed three different sequences from which you can choose, depending on your needs. The more regularly you are able to practice and the more time you can devote to it, the more benefits you will get from it. Practice the longest sequence as often as possible. However, even on those days when you are faced with a time crunch, you can squeeze in a short and effective practice. For those who do have the time and enthusiasm for an everyday practice, remember that it is always nice to give your body one day of rest per week.

Hold times. Please note that the timings for the poses are suggestions, rather than rules. In most poses, 1 minute is an average to aim for to get good results, but it may be too long at first if you have muscle weakness or intense sensation. Both of these will decrease with practice: muscles will strengthen and stretch, so that longer holds will be more comfortable; be patient and accept that 30 seconds may be sufficient to start with. As your experience and strength increase over time, you may want to challenge yourself with even longer holds of up to 2 minutes to build more strength. Some of the seated poses, such as Comfortable Seated Cross-Legged Pose (Sukhasana, Figure 2) and Hero's Pose (Virasana, Figure 12A or 12B), are commonly used for meditation and can be held for longer periods of time if desired, as long as there is no pain. Finally, in balance poses, it may be easier to count your breaths than to watch a clock or use a timer. This is especially true for Challenging Balance: Eyes Closed (Figure 7). In this case, try to keep your breath relaxed, slow, and steady, observing from within.

Knee Therapy Practice

45 minutes to 1 hour

For active rehabilitation, practice this longer sequence at least three or four times a week. Yoga is a daily practice, and every day is not too much for most of these poses, as long as you are gentle and attentive. An exception might be Hero's Pose (Virasana, Figure 12A or Figure 12B), which can be practiced on alternate days to start with if it is challenging.

Staff Pose: 30 seconds to 1 minute, Figure 1A or Figure 1B

Comfortable Seated Cross-Legged Pose: 30 seconds to 1 minute
per side, Figure 2

Cross-Legged Forward Bend Pose: 30 seconds to 1 minute, per side, Figure 3

Half-Dog Pose: 30 seconds to 1 minute, Figure 4

Seat-of-Power Pose: 30 seconds to 2 minutes, Figure 5

Tree Pose: 30 seconds to 1 minute, or 10 to 15 breaths, per side, Figure 6

Challenging Balance: Eyes Closed: 5 to 10 breaths, per side, Figure 7

Extended Triangle Pose: 30 seconds to 1 ½ minutes, per side, Figure 8A
or Figure 8B

Warrior II Pose: 30 seconds to 1½ minutes, per side, Figure 9

Warrior I Pose: 30 seconds to 1½ minutes, per side, Figure 10

Half-Frog Pose: 45 seconds, per side, Figure 11

Hero's Pose: 1 to 3 minutes, Figure 12A or Figure 12B

Downward-Facing Dog Pose: 30 seconds to 2 minutes, Figure 13

Thread the Needle I: 1 minute per side, Figure 14

Thread the Needle II: 30 seconds to 1½ minutes, per side, Figure 15A
or Figure 15B

Reclining Twist Pose: 1 minute, per side, Figure 16

Relaxation Pose: at least 10 minutes!, Figure 17

Healthy Knees Maintenance Practice

30 to 45 minutes

The reality of modern life is that most of us don't have the time for an hour of yoga every day of the year. The longer sequence can be practiced often, and at least every other day is recommended when you are actively rehabilitating your knees. Although it is important to keep up your yoga practice to maintain the healing benefits, eventually you can reduce your therapeutic program to two to three times a week. This shorter sequence can be alternated with the Knee Therapy Practice Sequence, and is useful for days when you have less time.

Staff Pose: 30 seconds to 1 minute, Figure 1A or Figure 1B

Comfortable Cross-Legged Seated Pose: 30 seconds to 1 minute, per side, Figure 2

Cross-Legged Forward Bend Pose: 30 seconds to 1 minute, per side, Figure 3

Tree Pose: 30 seconds to 1 minute, or 10 to 15 breaths, per side, Figure 6

Challenging Balance: Eyes Closed: 5 to 10 breaths, per side, Figure 7

Extended Triangle Pose: 30 seconds to 1½ minutes, per side, Figure 8A or 8B

Warrior II Pose: 30 seconds to 1½ minutes, per side, Figure 9

Half-Frog Pose: 45 seconds, per side, Figure 11

Downward-Facing Dog Pose: 30 seconds to 2 minutes, Figure 13

Thread the Needle I: 1 minute per side, Figure 14

Reclining Twist Pose: 1 minute per side, Figure 16

Relaxation Pose: 5 to 10 minutes!, Figure 17

The I-Don't-Have-Time-to-Practice Practice

15 to 20 minutes

Some days, we just don't have time to practice. But something is better than nothing, and taking 15 minutes to care for yourself on a busy day is a healthy habit to develop. Here are the poses you should try to fit in every day, and a sequence you can use on those days when time is especially short.

Seat-of-Power Pose: 30 seconds to 1 minute, repeat twice, Figure 5

Challenging Balance: Eyes Closed: 10 breaths, Figure 7

Thread the Needle I, Thread the Needle II, or both: 30 seconds to 1 minute, per side, Figure 14, Figure 15A, and Figure 15B

Half-Frog Pose, 45 seconds, per side, Figure 11

Half Downward-Facing Dog Pose or Downward-Facing Dog Pose: 1 minute, Figure 4 or Figure 13

Child's Pose: 1 minute, see page 63

Relaxation Pose: 5 minutes, Figure 17

Practice note: If you are too pressed for time to really relax in Relaxation Pose, instead just sit in Comfortable Seated Cross-Legged Pose (Figure 2), and focus on your breath for 10 slow, steady breaths. Then try revisit this relaxed breathing as you go about your day.

Part Three

Everyday Knees

▼ ▼ ▼ ▼ ▼ ▼ ▼ ▼ ▼ ▼ ▼ ▼ ▼

MANY OF US take our bodies for granted until something goes wrong. If you are not naturally physically inclined, you may unconsciously view your body simply as transportation, and neglect to care for its physical health. A naturally athletic person often places great—even unreasonable—demands on the body. Over time, either extreme leads to problems. Your body cannot be of continuous service without proper care, any more than your car can. If you neglect your car, eventually it will fall apart; if you abuse it, the engine will burn out. But at least a car can be replaced with a new model.

Just as your car needs regular maintenance to extend its life and keep it running efficiently, your body needs to be cared for. At a practical level, yoga, which takes the joints through their full range of motion and creates strong, supple muscles, is one valuable tool for caring for yourself holistically. Regular practice will help you move and live more consciously in your body. But even if you manage to practice yoga every day, that will not, by itself, compensate for neglect or abuse the rest of the time.

Knee problems are common because knees are one of the trickiest, most vulnerable parts of the body. It could be said that knees have an imperfect design: perhaps evolution is still working on the final model. In the meantime, this design is what we've got to work with. Accordingly, here are a few tips to give your knees a little extra support, so that they can continue to support you as you move through the world on your legs each day.

Shoes. Wear supportive, comfortable shoes. Take a look at the heels of the shoes you wear often. If the inner or outer heel is worn down, it's time to get rid of them. Then get fitted for shoes that are designed for your particular type of feet. There are great shoes designed specifically for pronation and supination control. If your problems are more severe or you can't find shoes that do the job, go to a podiatrist and get orthotic inserts for your shoes to help keep your feet and ankles in balance when you walk.

Be aware, however, that the science of orthotics is a profitable enterprise; investigate whether you actually have flat feet or if you can develop your arches through strengthening the supporting muscles. As someone who had collapsed arches, I can personally attest to the benefits of strengthening the feet and ankles. Although I will always have some natural tendency toward pronation, the difference my yoga practice made is dramatic. My shoes, which once wore down at the inner heels and no longer do, are tangible evidence of this.

Replace your shoes regularly, especially athletic shoes and shoes that you walk long distances in. Don't wear high heels, at least not for everyday. How your shoes feel and whether they are appropriate for your particular feet are far more important than how they look.

Feet. Go barefoot whenever you can. Our species didn't evolve wearing shoes. Although shoes are a great invention, both for protecting our feet from harsh environments and for fashion purposes, our feet and ankle muscles tend to be underdeveloped from wearing shoes all the time. This is why beginning students often experience cramps in their feet and ankle muscles when first learning standing poses; if the feet are always protected, they won't be accustomed to working to give you optimum support. At home, on the beach, or in grassy meadows, take off your shoes, enjoy being barefoot, and let the muscles of your feet do the work they are meant to.

Bring more awareness to how your feet function in everyday life: Practice lifting and spreading your toes, practice consciously walking on the four corners of your feet. Whether or not you have knee problems, creating more awareness and stability in the knee and ankle joints has many benefits, not the least of which is helping you maintain a good sense of balance as you age.

For athletes. Stretch immediately after your workout or sport—every time. Stretch your hips, quads, hamstrings, and calves. Athletic activity tightens these muscles considerably, and keeping them supple is essential for maintaining healthy knees. Stretching your muscles will not reduce their strength, and it will increase your range of motion, which can only be good for athletic performance. In addition, flexible muscles will keep your body youthful, allowing you to participate in your chosen activity longer and with fewer injuries.

Deep stretching is neither necessary nor advisable *before* working out, because cold joints and muscles are vulnerable to injuries and tears. Before a major workout, warm up slowly with mild aerobic activity. Afterward, when your muscles are warm and before they have tightened up, is when you will benefit from deeper stretching, and when it is most important. Don't skip the stretching portion of your workout, thinking you'll be going to yoga class later in the week anyway. If you don't have time on the field after your soccer game, at least take 15 or 20 minutes to stretch before going to bed that same night.

For those with a less-active lifestyle. Move! But move consciously and cautiously. If you haven't been exercising much, it will take some time for your muscles and joints to build strength and flexibility, so don't try to start with marathon running. Build up your level of activity slowly. Walking, swimming, tai chi, and Pilates are good complementary disciplines to yoga. And remember to stretch after your exercise sessions. It is normal to have sore muscles following any new physical activity, but if the soreness is too intense, it will be hard to stay motivated. Mild stretching will help reduce soreness. The sore-muscle phase is temporary if you keep at it. So find physical activities that you like enough to make them part of your life.

Knee injuries. If you have a knee injury or are recovering from one, avoid high impact activities, such as jogging, bowling, aerobics classes, and working out on some cardio gym equipment. Choose alternatives, such as walking, swimming, Pilates, tai chi, or working out on nonimpact gym equipment.

Bicycling is often recommended as a nonimpact exercise that strengthens the muscles of the knees. *Two caveats:* Although bicycling is therapeutic for some knee conditions, it is contraindicated for others. Your doctor is the best guide as to whether it can benefit your particular condition. (If you feel pain, bicycling is exacerbating, rather than healing, your injury. The downside of bicycling is how tight it makes your leg and hip muscles: a regular, thorough after-cycling stretching program is essential.

Moving from sitting to standing. Standing up after sitting in a chair can strain your knees, especially if you were sitting in a very low chair. Use your arms to help you stand up, rather than pushing entirely from your legs.

Do something you love every day. If you have joy in your life, you'll have more enthusiasm and energy for life, and less time for pain. Some of my greatest joy in life has come from my love of books, and I try to make regular time for reading throughout my week.

The Hatha Yoga Pradipika, attributed to Svatmarama (15th century A.C.E.), is the first known text specifically about Hatha Yoga. Subscribing to an admittedly liberal interpretation of the text, which advises that "needless austerities"[3] are an obstacle to practice, I also recommend not denying yourself small indulgences from time to time, such as a little chocolate or sneaking off for an afternoon movie. Think about what you personally enjoy the most—whether it's solitary time outdoors, being surrounded by children or by art, or an occasional day at a spa—and then make the space to have more pleasure in your life. Will it help your knees? It certainly won't hurt them! It is my experience that happiness is healing.

3. Svatmarama, *The Hatha Yoga Pradipika*, trans. Brian Dana Akers (Woodstock, N.Y.: YogaVidya, 2002), 6.

Yoga with Sandy Blaine

Alameda Yoga Station
1347 Park St., #D
Alameda, CA 94501
(510) 523-9642, www.alamedayogastation.com

The Yoga Room
2640 College Ave.
Berkeley, CA 94704
(510) 273-9273
www.yogaroomberkeley.com

For more information about her classes and workshops, you can e-mail Sandy Blaine at yogastat@aol.com. Please note that she cannot diagnose your condition, and cannot give you individual yoga advice about your knees by phone or e-mail.

Clothing and Props Photographed in Yoga for Healthy Knees

Props: Hugger-Mugger Yoga Products, (800) 473-4888, www.huggermugger.com

Clothing: Marie Wright Yoga Wear, (800) 217-0006, www.mariewright.com

Other Recommended Resources

BOOKS

Desikachar, T. K. V. *The Heart of Yoga: Developing a Personal Practice.* Rochester, Vt.: Inner Traditions, 1999.

Feuerstein, Georg. *The Shambhala Guide to Yoga: An Essential Introduction to the Principles and Practice of an Ancient Tradition.* Boston: Shambhala, 1996.

Lasater, Judith, Ph.D., P.T. *30 Essential Yoga Poses: For Beginning Students and Their Teachers.* Berkeley, Calif.: Rodmell Press, 2003.

———. *Living Your Yoga: Finding the Spiritual in Everyday Life.* Berkeley, Calif.: Rodmell Press, 2000.

McClure, Vimala. *A Woman's Guide to Tantric Yoga.* Novato, Calif.: New World Library, 1997.

Mehta, Mira. *How to Use Yoga: A Step-by-Step Guide to the Iyengar Method of Yoga, for Relaxation, Health, and Well-Being.* Berkeley, Calif.: Rodmell Press, 1998.

Mehta, Sylva, Mira Mehta, and Shayam Mehta. *Yoga: The Iyengar Way.* New York: Knopf, 1990.

Schiffman, Erich. *Yoga: The Art and Practice of Moving Into Stillness.* New York: Pocket, 1996.

Tomlinson, Cybèle. *Simple Yoga: A Simple Wisdom Book.* Berkeley, Calif.: Conari Press, 2000.

MAGAZINES

The following magazines have published articles by Sandy Blaine:

Ascent
www.ascentmagazine.com

Yoga International
www.yimag.org

Yoga Journal
www.yogajournal.com

WHERE TO FIND A YOGA TEACHER ONLINE

www.yogaalliance.com
www.yogajournal.com
www.yogateachersassoc.org

Ongoing public yoga classes are not geared toward rehabilitative yoga and cannot always be easily adapted for individual needs. If you have an acute knee problem, I recommend that you work with a qualified teacher on a one-to-one basis in order to set up an individual therapeutic yoga program, or look for workshops that address your particular condition.

About the Model

▼ ▼ ▼ ▼ ▼ ▼ ▼

Deborah Ramelli lives in the San Francisco Bay Area, where she has taught yoga classes and led retreats since 1996. She has traveled widely and studied extensively in her passionate pursuit of the path of yoga. Deborah loves sharing this passion with her students in her creative, informative, and nurturing classes. She is a student of Ramanand Patel and of Dr. K. L. S. Jois, of Mysore, India. Deborah is currently pursuing studies in holistic nutrition at Bauman College in Penngrove, California, as a way to help further empower her students to optimize their well-being.

For information about her classes, workshops, and retreats, e-mail her at dramelli@hotmail.com.

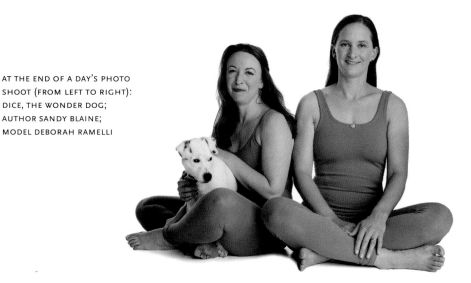

AT THE END OF A DAY'S PHOTO
SHOOT (FROM LEFT TO RIGHT):
DICE, THE WONDER DOG;
AUTHOR SANDY BLAINE;
MODEL DEBORAH RAMELLI

About the Author

▼ ▼ ▼ ▼ ▼ ▼ ▼

Sandy Blaine grew up in Berkeley, California, where she took her first yoga class in 1987, and immediately fell in love with its beauty and mystery. She has a joyous devotion to her own daily yoga practice, which she strives to share with her students through her teaching and her writing.

Sandy has been teaching yoga full time in the San Francisco Bay Area since 1993, where she got her start teaching at the University of California, Berkeley. In 1995, she graduated from the Advanced Studies Program at Berkeley's Yoga Room; she joined their faculty in 2000. She is one of the founders of the Alameda Yoga Station, which opened in 1995 and which she codirects. In addition to teaching her weekly classes in Berkeley and Alameda, she has been the in-house yoga teacher at Pixar Animation Studios in Emeryville, California, since 1994.

Sandy's writing has appeared in *Ascent, Yoga International,* and *Yoga Journal.* In 2004, she wrote a series on home practice, "Asana at Home," for *Yoga International's* "Asana" column. Her current writing projects include a book on developing a personal yoga practice and other Rodmell Press Yoga Shorts projects.

Sandy resides in Oakland, California, where, when not teaching, practicing, or writing about yoga, she enjoys reading, cooking, and hiking in the Oakland hills.

For more information about her yoga classes and workshops, visit www.alamedayogastation.com and www.yogaroomberkeley.com. You can e-mail her at yogastat@aol.com.

From the Publisher

▼ ▼ ▼ ▼ ▼ ▼ ▼

Rodmell Press publishes books on yoga, Buddhism, and aikido. In the Bhagavadgita it is written, "Yoga is skill in action." It is our hope that our books will help individuals develop a more skillful practice—one that brings peace to their daily lives and to the Earth.

We thank all whose support, encouragement, and practical advice sustain us in our efforts. In particular, we are grateful to Reb Anderson, B. K. S. Iyengar, Wendy Palmer, and Yvonne Rand for their inspiration.

To request a catalog or be on our e-announcements list, contact us at:

(510) 841-3123

(800) 841-3123

(510) 841-3191 (fax)

info@rodmellpress.com

www.rodmellpress.com

Rodmell Press is distributed to the trade by Publishers Group West:

(800) 788-3123

(510) 528-5511 (sales fax)

info@pgw.com

Index

▼ ▼ ▼ ▼ ▼ ▼ ▼